BLOOD TYPE DIET MISTAKES TO AVOID: A SIMPLIFIED GUIDE TO AVOID COMMON MISTAKES FOR BLOOD TYPE O, A, AB & B

EMILY FAN 2017 All Rights Reserved

WITHDRAWN

The facts herein provided is truthful in all its entirety and coherent, in that no legal responsibility, in the form of consideration or else by the use or misuse of any strategies, procedures or directions contained within shall lie against the author such liability thereon is the sole and the utter obligation of the reader solely. Under no situation will any legal duty or blames be imputed or held out unfavorable the publisher(s) for any form of compensation, damages, pecuniary loss due to the information contained herein be it direct or indirect.

The guide, direction, material, and instructions that are offered here is for the purposes of information only and is universal as such. The information presented here is without any form of contract or guarantee or indemnity whether with the reader or any third party.

INTRODUCTION

Congratulations for downloading this book. No matter how many books that you have read on the blood type diet, no matter how long you have been on the blood type diet, you cannot succeed in the diet and lose weight if you make mistakes that are avoidable.

Through this book, you will learn the essential mistakes that you need to avoid in the blood type diet and what to do to avoid those mistakes effortlessly.

TABLE OF CONTENTS

INTRODUCTION	**3**
PART 1	**1**
MISTAKE1#: THE PATH OF RESISTANCE	**1**
MISTAKE2#: LONE RANGER	**6**
PART 2	**9**
MISTAKE3#: THE PATH OF RECIPES	**9**
MISTAKE4#: DIETING WITHOUT A MAP	**15**
MISTAKE5#: JUNK ERROR	**20**
MISTAKE6#: THE BUDGET TEARS	**22**
PART 3	**35**
MISTAKE7#: KEEPING AN EYE ON THE SCALE	**35**

MISTAKE8#: EATING PHOBIA	**39**
MISTAKE9#: CHEAT DAYS THAT KILLS	**41**
MISTAKE10#: YOU'RE STUBBORN	**43**
MISTAKE11#: YOU ARE NOT REALLY IN	**45**

PART 4   48

MISTAKE12#: MIRACLE SOLUTIONS	**48**
MISTAKE13#: MEDICATION THAT CAN BE A CULPRIT	**50**
MISTAKE14#: THE SECRET OF STRESS FOR YOUR TYPE	**51**
MISTAKE15#: EXERCISE SLIP	**56**

PART 5   60

MISTAKE16#: GOING OVER BOARD	**60**
MISTAKE17#: QUICK TO QUIT	**62**
MISTAKE18#: FAILURE TO INDIVIDUALIZED YOUR PLAN	**64**
MISTAKE19#: WHEN OTHERS BECOME YOUR GUIDE	**66**

MISTAKE 20#: DIVERSITY THAT SPICE THE DIET	**69**
MISTAKE 21#: SUPPLEMENTS SHORT COMING	**71**

PART 6	**76**

MISTAKE 22#: HIDDEN DIET STRATEGIES	**76**
MISTAKE 23#: DOUBT THAT DESTROY	**82**
MISTAKE # 24: THE 100 METRES DASH RACE	**87**
MISTAKE #25: THE JOURNAL ACCIDENT	**89**
OTHER BOOKS BY THE SAME AUTHOR	**92**

PART 1

Mistake1#: The Path of Resistance

The blood type diet has gone through a lot of period of tempestuous waves before gaining the popularity it now enjoys. Before I proceed, I would love to lay down some background information on the blood type diet.

Blood Type Diet Mistakes to Avoid

The blood type diet was founded by Naturopath, Dr. Peter J. Adamo who inherited the work from his father. The basis of the research is that one man's food is another man's poison. This is rooted in the blood group of each individual that what one person loves, another may hate it. The different blood groups of O, A, B, and AB have foods that they flourish on based on their original make up. When a person who does not observe this medical injunction eats everything that he wants, a compendium of problems descends on the person. The food that blood type A eats cannot be the same as the food that blood type O eats. Essentially, there are antigens in the blood and the food that humans consume. When these antigens react with the food that people eat, they cause a variety of problems such as diseases, health complication, etc.

In the early days of the diet, there was a lot of controversies that surrounded its scientific foundation. Many people claimed that the diet could not be supported by valid and scientifically proven results. Although these arguments have all been laid to a final interment, there are still some small dissidents who have hurdled up and strew internet materials canvassing arguments against the diet.

The intent of this book is not to join issues with these people. They can hold onto their arguments while those who are interested in the diet that has become the solace for weight loss for over 7 million people around the world can continue to diet in peace. Real evidence of weight loss destroys arguments.

As a dieter, whether seasoned or a beginner, you will still follow this path of resistance. There are various obstacles in the blood type diet, and they present themselves at different stages of the diet. Some of this resistance could come from family members who will despise your diet and still find reasons to tell you that the diet will not work. Others are friends, and in some cases, you can be your own problem. You can stumble and fall. Make mistakes but correct them as soon you discover where you have fallen. The resistance and trial of your diet will come in many formats. Your body may protest because of the changes that you have made. Remember that you have been eating just about what you feel like eating for a long time. But whatever form the mistakes may take, I have provided a solid information on how to deal with those mistakes. I will explain them one after the other and the solutions to each of these mistakes.

Mistake2#: Lone Ranger

Every diet has its own challenges. They each have their difficulties which the dieter must overcome. These problems will become overpowering when you walk the path of the blood type diet alone. In this days of internet flexibility and globalization, you can be in Manhattan while someone in Houston, Texas is offering you valuable help.

There are many social media interactive pages, Facebook groups, twitter, etc., that offer blood type diet support. You can join these groups and see how some blood type dieters are faring in the diet. No challenge that you are going to be confronted with in the blood type diet is new. From finding recipes to cooking to shopping, to supplements and reactions that you physically see on your body, nothing is new to other dieters. The challenge that you are facing which is threatening to kick you out of the diet is what someone has experienced and successfully overcome. All that you need to do is ask for some help, and people will be glad to help you.

Besides, there are diverse online forums for your blood type that are able to proffer solutions for your type. Join them and receive help. In this global age of digitalization, you can't walk alone. Look for support groups and become a part of them. It is through these groups that you will be able to receive the help that you need.

PART 2

Mistake3#: The path of Recipes

If you are reading this book right now, I assume that you have already known your blood type. So I will skip this. But if you do not know your blood type, I will suggest that you go for a blood type test. It is simple. That will give you a head start as to how to begin the blood type diet. Additional, you can look at this book for a simplified 5-step procedure on how to begin the blood type diet (BLOOD TYPE DIET FOR O & A: A SIMPLIFIED BEGINNERS APPROACH TO EATING RIGHT FOR YOUR BLOOD TYPE - Kindle edition by Emily Fan. Cookbooks, Food & Wine Kindle eBooks @ Amazon.com. and Amazon.com: BLOOD TYPE DIET FOR AB & B: What Every Beginner Must Know to Lose Weight eBook: Emily Fan: Kindle Store .) These two books are free in the kindle store.

Whatever blood type you belong to, there are different foods to eat and avoid. This basic knowledge is non-negotiable for beginning the blood type diet and for those who have been on the diet. The basic knowledge or generic information that patents into your diet are important. In other words, what am I supposed to know as blood type O, A, AB, and B? When you have this basic knowledge about your blood type, then you will avoid the mistakes that some people on the blood type diet make.

Let's attempt a simplified explanation of the blood type diet. According to Dr. Peter J. Adamo, Blood type O should eat low-carb and high protein. They will eat mostly meat and fish. They are also not to eat dairy products as this may cause problems for them because of their blood type. Their diet consists of beef, turkey, and fruits, but they are to limit dairy products. They are to avoid oranges, avocado, and pork amongst others.

For blood type A, they are primarily vegetarians, and they are to eat mostly vegetables. They are however to limit the intake of chicken and turkey as D' Adamo has recommended. If blood type A violates this dieting rules, they will experience weight gain. The blood type A suffers from acute shortage of acidic stomach content.

They have the inability to digest protein derived from meat, particularly red meat.

For Type B, D' Adamo recommended that they should eat certain types of meats, fish and dairy products and then eat plenty of vegetables. They, however, must avoid the consumption of turkey, chicken, pork, and poultry.

Blood Type AB is a blend of A and B has a varied food to eat. He endorsed for them to eat – fish, turkey, yogurt, soft cheese, nuts, and beans. They are however to ensure the avoidance of the following foods – pork, corn, bell peppers and black olives.

From the above simple explanation, you can see that each of the food blood types have their own type of food. A good dieter will avoid these mistakes by fortifying himself with this basic knowledge.

Even when you have armed yourself with this information, there are certain things which you've to do. A blood type diet is a unique form of eating. It has highly beneficial recipes, recipes to avoid and neutral recipes. As a dieter, you may need to have some basic knowledge about these foods that you are to eat, avoid and neutral ones. I am not saying go over to the recipes for your type and memorize them. No, that is not what I mean. Just a simple glance at the food list for your type will be more than sufficient. Once you are equipped with this rudimentary knowledge, you are able to diet without having to skip the recipes which you are supposed to eat.

Mistake4#: Dieting without a map

You have heard this popular saying that if you fail to plan, you have plan to fail. This is true in all respect. To succeed in the blood type diet, you need to have a concrete plan. A map of recipes. And consistently update your plan in order to keep on enjoying your diet. Dieting without a map or meal plan is one of the biggest mistakes of many dieters. Majority of the members of the blood type diet who do not plan end up failing entirely. Although planning may take your time, when you do that, you are saved from a lot of trouble that may arise. Knowing what to eat at a particular time, help you to prepare for a healthy life of dieting. Some people cheat on the blood type diet because they do not have a meal plan. They binge here and there and eat food that may end up affecting their health and weight. Let us consider the various benefits of having a good plan.

There are several reasons why you need a diet plan to ensure that you lose weight effortlessly. Let us now consider some of the reasons why you actually need a diet plan.

First, having a meal plan gives you the certainty of what foods you are to eat. The beauty of this is that it tells you with accurate precision the food that you are to eat daily. What you are to eat for breakfast, lunch, and dinner are prepared. You will not need to start thinking about what you are to eat for breakfast or dinner since your meal plan is already prepared. Thus, this guarantees the foods to eat per day and during the week. This is one of the interesting reasons why you need a diet plan as a beginner or pro.

Flexibility. When you have prepared a meal plan, you can change your diet whenever you desire. Once you discover certain foods that can make your blood type diet interesting within your beneficial foods list, you can change it at any time.

A meal helps you to stay organized. With a meal plan, your diet is organized. You can make use of a computer spreadsheet or an android or IOS app for planning your meals. Then you can organize what you are to eat in a day. You can decide to do a 14 days meal plan or 7 days meal plan.

Through a meal plan, you will know precisely the things that you are to buy for your dieting. A simple or casual look at your meal plan will reveal to you the things that you will need to purchase at the grocery store.

Mistake5#: Junk Error

The blood type diet is a highly restrictive diet that tells you the food that you are supposed to eat and the foods that you are supposed to avoid. The blood type diet centres on eating whole food and real food. When you become a fan of processed foods, then the blood type diet will be hard for you to carry out. All the foods that are recommended for your blood type are natural foods that have not been processed. The advantage of eating natural foods are myriad. Buying organic food is the best option that a blood type dieter should choose. Besides being the healthiest choice for rapid weight loss, it is not fraught with the danger of pesticide contamination which is often the case for non-organic-based foods. One of the mistakes of the blood type diet is when you keep eating processed food. You will not only be breaching the rules of the diet, but you may also be eating food that is not blood type diet compliant. Then the problem of weight gain and health becomes apparent.

The best type of food that human beings have been used to for millions of years are organic or whole food. But when industrial revolution kicks in, the man began to deviate from natural foods to planting and processing. Today, many stores are lined up with processed foods on their shelves. However, the blood type diet recommends food that is organic, in their natural state. Oils, vegetables, nuts, seafood, etc., are food that is organic in nature.

Mistake6#: The Budget Tears

Have you seen the blood type diet recipes recommended for your type? Have your perused through the entire food that your blood type as O, A, B, and AB is supposed to eat? What did you realize? All the foods are natural foods! You are right! And this is one of the biggest mistakes of many blood type dieters. They commenced the diet thinking that all is going to be easy on their budget and pocket. You will spend money on the recipes that you are to eat on the blood type diet. Recipes for unprocessed foods are expensive.

Some dieters get kicked out of the blood type diet because of the expensive recipes. I have taken time to explain how to ovoid this big mistake in two of my books Amazon.com: BLOOD TYPE DIET FOR BEGINNERS: Eat Right For Your Blood Type With O, A, B And

AB Negative eBook: Emily Fan: Kindle Store and Amazon.com: BLOOD TYPE DIET FOR BEGINNERS: Your Guide To Eat Right 4 Your Type And Lose Up To A Pound A Day: Lose Weight Fast, Look Healthy With Your Blood Type O, A, B And AB eBook: EMILY FAN: Kindle Store. But let me further explain to you the simple ways to avoid this mistake that many of the blood type dieters are making.

Dirty Dozen Tool

The Environmental Working Group has over the years developed a list of non-organic foods that are least affected by pesticides. Even though this list fluctuates all the time because of the research which the organization carries out, you can rely on this list for buying non-organic foods which are almost chemical free. The fruits are organized in descending order. Those with the most amount of pesticides start from number 1 while those with a lower amount of pesticides are from number 51 below. Some of the fruits and veggies in the dirty dozen lists Shoppers Guide to Pesticides are:

• Carrots

- Oranges

- Green Onions

- Watermelon

- Grapefruit

- Eggplant

- Pineapple

You can check the complete list on their website at www.ewg.org/foodnews/list.php.

The dirty dozen tool is a great way to reduce the cost of blood type diet.

Let nothing be wasted! It will help you to cut down cost. This is the most efficient way to manage resources. For instance, the bones you have used are not to be discarded; you can reuse them for making another set of broth. The pan drippings you used can be reserved for later use. For your fresh produce, employ wisdom. Do not waste it. Cut just about what you need. Throw nothing away.

Waste Nothing.

Food wastage is one of the biggest problems of dieters – whether they are veteran dieters or beginners. Food wastage will draw many holes in your wallet and finances. Your leftovers should not be a bosom friend of the dustbin. It should be frozen in the refrigerator to be used again. A food saver will help you to save money. Your vegetables may not look freshly appetizing from 3 days ago, but they are still delicious with nutritional value. So don't waste any of your food. It will make your low budget blood type diet a reality.

Direct Farmers Purchase

The farmers market that is near you is a great source of fresh and inexpensive food. Once you identify yourself with the local farmers around you, it will amaze you the amount of money that you will save when you have a personal relationship with the local farmers, and you begin to buy fresh produce directly from them.

Bulk Purchase

One of the easiest ways to save money is to purchase your food items in bulk. For instance, a bag of chicken in a nearby store around you can be $ 10 and can last you almost a week. For those who want to shop online, check for Grassland Beef that can be shipped to your house in a frozen box. The great thing about bulk buying is that it gives a discount that you will not be able to get if you buy your items one after the other. If the goods that you want to purchase are seasonal goods, then during the season make your purchases in large quantity. If you buy in bulk, you can preserve the freshness of your product by either freezing, fermenting or other methods of preservation that is best suited to you.

Home-Made stuff

If you buy everything you need for your blood type diet, it will increase your expenses. However, if you make your own flavour, expenses on the blood type would be minimized. Prepare your homemade stock and other condiments that you make by yourself. This will reduce expenses. Let this be a discipline that you will learn every time by making your own stuff from scratch. What you need if you want to make everything yourself are the basic ingredients.

Costco Membership

This is one of my favourites. Aimed at cutting down the cost of your blood type diet, then you may consider Costco membership or any membership at your local food store or market. Get a Costco membership card. The membership card for gold card owners will cost you an amazing $ 55 per year. There is another membership card that cost $ 110 per year. Depending on your financial weight, you can get a membership card and enjoy a lot of discounts. A complete rotisserie chicken will cost you $ 5, and they are very big, and two dozen of eggs cost just $ 3. These rotisserie chickens contain no extra fat, or preservatives, gluten, non-natural flavours or colors. There are other inexpensive items when purchased in bulk such as oils, nuts, avocado, meat, and cheese. Depending on your blood type, you can buy these items in bulk. This will help you to save a lot of money and cut down the cost of your blood type diet. If you live in the UK, Costco in London is three – Chingford, Thurrock, and Wardford. If you live in Germany, you can find Costco in Berlin, Frankfurt, and Hussen. In Australia, you can find Costco in Docklands, Canberra, Auburn, and Adelaide. Besides that, you can do a simple Google search of Costco near you.

Buy Inexpensive Blood Type Diet Recipes

Have you seen the price of organic recipes in the store? Expensive huh? Yes, they are and to lower the cost of your Blood type diet, buy inexpensive recipes. Buy simple recipes like meat, seasonal veggies, nuts, and cheese.

To avoid the blood type diet being too expensive, find ways to cut down the cost of dieting by following simple wisdom plans.

PART 3

Mistake7#: Keeping an Eye on the Scale

One noticeable hallmark of the blood type diet is that it can help you lose a lot of weight within a very short time. The success stories of the blood type diet which you heard from people or read about from the internet may have influenced your decision to begin the diet.

Since you were wooed to the blood type diet by weight loss, you keep a constant eye on the scale. Always checking to see the number of pounds that you have dropped. There is nothing wrong with checking your weight, but if you climb the weight scale all the time, it can become a problem. It begins to burn down your motivation. Thoughts like I should have lost 3 pounds now, but I only lost 1 will begin to set in. Do not lose hope when you notice that your expectations are not met as they should. The best thing to do is to get on the scale before you begin the blood type diet. You can also measure your weight by measuring the circumference of your waist with a tape to know your weight. Know that your weight may be inconsistent depending on the stability of fluids and what is contained in your stomach. That is why you must not become a scale watcher constantly going on the scale to check the scale. You should check your scale at least three to four times in a month. Do it wisely. The blood type diet is a lifestyle and a healthy way of eating not just eating to lose weight.

For weight loss, have a moderate expectation. Aim towards 1 to 2 pounds in the first week of dieting. Then try to focus on losing 1 pound weekly. Then progress with it gradually. But when your expectation is too big, and they are not met, discouragement sets in and you are like, this diet does not work as people have said. Weight loss in young men tends to be faster than in older women.

Sometimes, you may feel that your weight loss has stopped. This could take weeks or days. Do not be moved by your physical appearance. When this happened, continue dieting and do not allow that to be a source of distraction.

You need to know that physical changes take time to appear.

Mistake8#: Eating Phobia

The blood type diet is not a fasting diet. You do not need to starve yourself because you want to lose weight. Other diets may allow that, but the blood type diet does not allow that. You do not have to remain hungry because you are pursuing weight loss. Weight loss in the blood type diet comes naturally once you are able to eat according to your blood type. Whether blood type O, A, AB, and B, each of the diet has a particular manner of eating that has been prescribed for you. The blood type diet recipes are weight loss recipes. Whether you are eating because the clock says so or you are eating because you are hungry, do not be afraid to eat. In the blood type diet, you do not have to be scared of foods that are structured according to your blood type. When you starve yourself, cravings can occur, and the desire to eat what does not belong to your type can be overpowering. The best thing to do is to consume foods in your type as frequently as you desire to eat. No starvation. It is a blood type diet, not a starvation diet. So you have to eat when you are hungry or when the need for food arises.

Mistake9#: Cheat Days that Kills

If you have been following the blood type diet for a while now, you might be feeling that cheating occasionally will do you no harm. However, this attitude is a diet sabotage. It hinders your weight loss and may cause other forms of health complications. Even the smallest amount of food that is not based on your blood type can prevent you from losing weight. It is possible that you might feel bad for turning down a piece of red meat as a type A or as type O, turning down a cup of latte someone invited you for a cup might be difficult. That is true. You have to understand that for every little cheat days that you contemplate or allow, you take yourself backward and jeopardize your weight loss and healthy lifestyle. It is like getting on the blood type diet today and going out of the diet tomorrow. That is what cheat days do to you. It is one of the biggest mistakes which you must avoid completely.

If someone is inviting you over for lunch, it is advisable to look out for restaurants that support blood type diet friendly foods. If you do not know of any around your area, Google blood type diet friendly restaurants. With technology, it is possible to see the menu of the restaurant that you are going to visit. In order not to make a mistake about the recipes the restaurant, pick diets menu that are for your type and not for other blood types.

Mistake10#: You're Stubborn

The blood type diet is eating for your type not eating for our type. In fact, from the original inception of the research that led to the blood type diet, Peter J. Adamo's father started on the premises of One Man's food is another Man's Poison. This means that even though you are all blood type O or A, the reaction to the changes in the blood type diet might be different. Changing dietary habit is like trying to break free from addiction. While you struggle to make yourself free, your body will start reacting.

Besides, there are foods that may cause reactions in your body. Determine your allergy. No one may be telling you this, but it is because of this kind of mistake that many people have quit the blood type diet. The recipes for this diet are broken down into:

1. Highly Beneficial Recipes
2. Neutral Recipes
3. Recipes to Avoid

From these recipes, it is possible to discover that your body is reacting to the neutral recipes. Do not just shut your eyes and believe that everything is okay. You have to pay attention to your body. You can check each of the neutral recipes and see how your body responds to them for a possible allergy.

Mistake11#: You are not really in

A half-hearted commitment to the blood type diet will bring you no result in the blood type diet. This is an essential mistake to avoid. You are either in or not in at all. You can't be half in. But you must be really in. I mean totally in the diet and keep its rules. If you are not really in, the smallest form of trial or rejection will throw you out of the blood type diet. You are making a big shift in your diet, and it comes at a huge cost. A full commitment is needed to sustain your blood type diet eating habit.

Your diet will work well when you give it your all. Be committed and be faithful to the requirement of the blood type diet so that you can experience real changes. When the changes that you are expecting delays, your commitment will keep you going and moving forward. You should not be half in or sit on the fence in the blood type diet. You need a full fledge commitment to see results in the blood type diet.

PART 4

Mistake12#: Miracle Solutions

I know some of the people reading this book right now might have tried different diets. Many of them may have failed you. Having experienced repeated failures in different diets, you decided to try the blood type diet as a last resort. But do not look for the blood type diet as a miracle or quick fix solution.

Realistically, every diet that you undertake takes time to produce results. You can't begin the blood type diet today and see miraculous results tomorrow. It has to be gradual. Any diet that promises you instant result will remain at best a fad diet.

The blood type diet is not a quick fix solution to weight loss. To me, and I know you will soon agree with me, the blood type diet is a lifestyle. You make the changes that are necessary for lifestyle and healthy living and not just for some quick disappearing pounds. You need to put more effort towards a lifestyle than looking for a quick fix solution to your weight loss.

Mistake13#: Medication that can be a culprit

Never begin the blood type diet without consulting your physician if you are on medication. There are many drugs that can affect your weight loss. Some drugs can cause weight gain. . Certain antidepressants, heart burn drugs, corticosteroids, epilepsy drugs, and antibiotics cause weight gain. If you are on drugs, it is good to consult with your physician so that if the drugs that were prescribed for you can cause weight gain, you can know what to do. Dieting to lose weight and taking drugs that can cause weight gain is counterproductive measure. You will not lose weight even though you are on the blood type diet.

Mistake14#: The Secret of Stress for Your type

This is another huge mistake in the blood type diet that must be avoided. If you have begun the blood type diet and you have not been losing weight, it is time to stop and ask yourself some questions. Are you stress and do you try to rest when it is necessary? The human body has been designed to handle stress through a rather natural means.

Stress can hinder your weight loss in the blood type diet. Stress is a physical reaction which the body carries out when faced with difficult situations such as danger. When the body is stressed, it triggers a release of chemical materials such as cortisol, adrenaline, and norepinephrine in response to the stress that has occurred. Now when these chemical substances have been released into the blood system, and they are not cleared, they will cause weight gain.

For blood type O, when stress occurs, they have higher chances of gaining weight than blood type A. Blood type O does not quickly clear the stress hormone that has been pumped into the body system.

When stressed, Blood type A experience a rise in the presence of cortisol, a stress hormone known for causing weight gain. More than any other blood type, type A is plague by cortisol than blood type O, B, and AB. When situations that cause stress arises, type A produces more cortisol for handling the stress situation.

Blood type AB responds to stress just like type A. For type AB to effectively deal with stress, they need calming relaxation techniques such as low impact exercises.

For blood type B, their stress respond is similar to type A, and they share a common problem. Blood type B overproduce the hormone called cortisol which promotes weight gain. If you are type B and you are concerned about the rate of your weight loss, one of the things which you must check for is stress.

Solution to Stress

There are different forms of relaxation that have been put forward for different blood types of O, A, AB, and B. The blood type diet does not work on its own. Indeed, there are several factors that combine to make you lose weight including keeping your diet rules, eating regularly, etc. Simple relaxation techniques for your blood type, resting well and having some nice sleep help in dealing with stress. When you are not busy, sleeping early has been proven to be a good strategy for handling stress in the blood type diet.

Mistake15#: Exercise slip

The blood type diet is a unique diet. Each of the blood type of O, A, AB, and B have different forms of exercise that that they are supposed to do. To do an exercise that is not recommended for your blood type is a blood type diet common mistakes which must be avoided.

For instance, blood type O known for their rigorous strength and agility, have the capacity of their ancestors. They thrive on intense exercise. The type O does very well on serious exercises like a workout, swimming, cycling and any exercise that is rigorous. In sports, they are also excellent sportsmen and women. Sports such as basketball, soccer, and hockey suits them.

The best exercise for type A is relaxing and calm exercises. These physical activities will help them in maintaining a very balanced mind and body. When they exercise, the level of stress hormones in their body is reduced. Tai Chi, stretching, Pilates, dancing, rope skipping, gymnastics, and walking works well for blood type A.

Blood type B exercise is simple such as Aqua spinning, Ai chi, golf, tennis, Tai Chi, rowing, rope skipping and dancing. Type B exercise must be a workout that is low in intensity and resistance training.

For blood type AB, they can fit in the exercise of both A and B blood type. Their exercises are calm, relaxing and gentle such as hiking, walking, dancing or even golf. Tai chi is therapeutic for an AB type. When Type AB negative exercises, their stress hormones is reduced like adrenaline and cortisol.

Failure to exercise according to your blood type may result in weight gain since some of these exercises can trigger stress and cause weight gain. For example, if blood type A does exercise for type O, stress will occur, and the result will be weight gain.

PART 5

Mistake16#: Going over board

Although the blood type diet is highly restrictive, it allows for some form of freedom within the diet itself provided that the freedom is within the food recommended for your blood type. There are some foods that you can eat in moderation. For instance, blood type A can eat turkey and chicken as beneficial food recipes. This is a beneficial food; if type A eats chicken and turkey in excess, a problem will be created. Blood type A does not have the acidic stomach content necessary for digesting protein obtained from red meat. Another example is blood type O. Blood type are meat eaters. They can eat a lot of red meat and have no problem with eating. They are permitted, as a matter of freedom to eat certain types of beans in moderation. Let us look at going overboard for blood type O. If a blood type O decides to eat beans excessively because beans are permitted as neutral food or beneficial food, weight gain is already looming for that particular individual. The blood type O do not have the bacteria and enzymes that break down protein gotten from beans and plants. These two examples are clear cases of going overboard. When you do this, you are falling for one of the mistakes to avoid for your blood type. It will hinder effective weight loss.

Mistake17#: Quick to Quit

There is no place for quitters in anything in life. This is one of the common mistakes to avoid in the blood type diet if you want to achieve great results. Too many people quit on the verge of victory. They quit when results are about to start pouring in. It took you years of eating the wrong food to gather all the weight that you have now, and you want to lose it in a single day or week. If the weight took time to build, it would also take some time to be reduced.

Be Patient with the diet and with your body. The diet works and will give you the shape that you desire. However, it will be gradual as you drop those extra pounds of weight accumulated over a long period of time.

Mistake18#: Failure to Individualized your Plan

The blood type diet is eating for your type. Even if you are the same blood type O or A, there can never be an eating that fits all the members of the same blood group. There is no universal plan for the members of the same blood group. What works for another person may not work for you. Develop an eating plan that is well suited to you and not according to what someone has been doing. It is possible to hear some people say that they have found a diet plan that is suited for majority of them, but it may not work for you. Create a diet that suits you. You should have determined your allergy from the neutral recipes and customize your diet so that you can eat according to your type. It is possible that you and a friend share the same blood group, but you may have some allergies which he does not have. To share his diet plan will be to ignore your allergies and frustrate your diet.

So you have to make a diet plan that fits you. General diet plans can be a problem because they do not meet unique features of individual dieters in the blood type diet.

Mistake19#: When others become Your Guide

The body mechanism of everyone is different. Two people might be exposed to the same condition, yet the results from each of those persons may be different. That is the reason why you should not compare the results of your dieting with anyone. The blood type diet is guaranteed for weight loss. But the results of some in the diet should not become your guide. Each person may see a different outcome from the same diet. You may start the blood type diet on the same day with a fellow blood type O. However, your friend may see rapid weight loss within two weeks of commencing the diet.

When you begin to draw a comparison with the other individual, you are soon discouraged and may even quit the diet on the wrong belief that it is not working. You have to understand your body. Even if you are twins, I mean identical twins, from the same blood type A, the results that you will see in the blood type diet may be different. Each individual is not same. Salient differences among members of the same group abound.

While some people may experience common results with others such as weight loss, allergy to neutral recipes. That another person removed all those extra pounds in one week does mean that you too should expect the same result. If someone loss 2 pounds in a week, it does not mean that you will see the same result.

While some people may experience common results with others such as weight loss, allergy to neutral recipes, others may not. That another person removed all those extra pounds in one week does not mean that you too should expect the same result.

If someone loss 2 pounds in a week, it does not mean that you will see the same result.

Blood type diet results are affected by many factors even among the same blood type O, and A or among the same blood type B and AB. You should concentrate on achieving success for your diet than unnecessary comparison with others which will not help you in the blood type diet.

Mistake20#: Diversity that spice the diet

The monotony of the blood type diet is one of the common mistakes that must be avoided. You do not have to eat just one type of meal. When I mean diversify, I do not mean just eating veggies, fruits, etc. It is beyond that. To enjoy diversity, you should have a good understanding of your recipes. The recipes for your type.

Build a diet that allows you the freedom to eat every beneficial food for your blood type. Except if you have an allergy, you should be able to eat different foods for your blood type.

When the diet is arranged along some few recipes, it is possible to get tired of eating. As soon as this happens, the dieter may begin to eat foods not endorsed for his blood type. It won't be long before the individual gets kick out of the blood type diet. So eat everything for your blood type that is beneficial or neutral provided allergies don't affect you.

Mistake21#: Supplements Short coming

This is one of the mistakes that can be avoided in the blood type diet. If you are dieting without taking blood type diet supplements, you are missing some needful nutrients for your blood type.

Blood Type Diet Mistakes to Avoid

The blood type diet is a highly restrictive diet. It commands a way of eating that may exclude other vital nutrients out of your diet. During the time of dieting, nutritional needs become higher. Some nutrients which you should have eaten that your body needs are kept out because it is not according to your blood type. Since the diet cuts down on some fruits, veggies, and others, you may be missing some essential nutrients. That is the reason why you need to take blood type diet supplements.

The blood type diet recommends buying foods that are unprocessed or whole foods or organic foods. It can be by direct purchase from the farmers market that is near you. Though the foods are organic, this does not remove the needs for blood type diet supplements. Many of these farmers have farmed the lands intensively which prevent the nutrients from replenishing themselves through a natural means. When you buy your blood type diet recipes from farmers or organic food stores, it is possible for the foods that you have purchased to lack essential nutrients. That is the reason why you need to have supplements for your blood type. Other factors such as the inability of modern fertilizers to give sufficient nutrients to plants, the use of pesticides, transporting foods for a long distance, etc., are some of the reasons why you still need blood type diet supplements so that you can get the missing nutrients from your diet.

If you are blood type O, you can check out this book BLOOD TYPE DIET: EAT RIGHT FOR YOUR BLOOD TYPE FOOD AND SUPPLEMENTS FOR TYPE O - Kindle edition by EMILY FAN for your supplements.

If you are blood type A, check out this BLOOD TYPE DIET: EAT RIGHT FOR YOUR BLOOD TYPE FOOD AND SUPPLEMENTS FOR TYPE A - Kindle edition by EMILY FAN book for your supplement needs.

PART 6

Mistake22#: Hidden Diet Strategies

If you follow the diet plan, observe all of the rules of the blood type diet, but you do not know the hidden strategies for your type, you will not lose weight. Each of the blood types of O, A, AB, and B have a strategy that guarantees weight loss. So you have to know the strategy for your blood type for weight loss to be achieved.

If a blood type O must use noodles for recipes, it must be wheat free. There are many of them out there in the store. This simple formula will help you: What you can't digest plus diet will be equals to weight gain. As blood type O, you can't lose weight if you do not keep gluten and wheat out of your diet.

Type O are meat eaters. But it has been proven that lean meat for blood type O offers better diet results than conventional red meat. Lean meats such as turkey, chicken or beef encourage weight loss. Grass fed and not grain fed animals are suitable for you as type O.

As blood type O, they suffer from one inherent weakness – the shortage of iodine which controls the normal functioning of your thyroid. The thyroid helps in digestion, and you remember our earlier formula that indigestion is proportionally equaled to weight gain. An abnormal thyroid is the first step towards weight gain for blood type O. Seafood and iodized salt is recommended for blood type O in order to ensure a proper functioning thyroid.

For blood type A to avoid weight gain, lean turkey and chicken is okay if it is eaten in moderation. Your diet strategy lies in avoiding red meat since there is no acidic content in your stomach that will digest it.

You are a vegetarian by genetic makeup so you will be obtaining the majority of your protein needs from plants and leguminous crops.

For blood type AB, avoid red meat because of digestion problems so that you do not add extra pounds of weight and make your blood type diet ineffective. Avoid food that can prevent the normal functioning of your metabolism. You can digest yogurt and dairy products, but buckwheat interferes with metabolism so stay away from it. You have a sensitive stomach that reacts negatively to orange so watch out for it.

Type B hidden secrets for dieting that help them avoid common mistakes is to stay away from buckwheat. Dairy products do not constitute a problem for your type.

The consumption of lean meat such as lamb and venison is encouraged. However, red meat is a source of weight gain due to the poor acidic stomach content of blood type B. Eat oatmeal and millet moderately. Food for weight loss includes seafood, salmon, halibut, flounder, beets, and carrots.

Avoid the following foods so that you do not add weight as type B:

- Sesame seeds,
- Peanuts,
- Sunflower seeds.

Mistake 23#: Doubt that Destroy

The blood type diet is no fad diet. It has been subjected to the scientific test, and the diet works. Now, one of the mistakes of dieters especially beginners is the doubts on the efficacy of the diet. There are many arguments for and against the diet. Beyond the controversial arguments, does the diet works? Has there been any report emanating from any source that the diet has negatively impacted the health of the dieter? Instead of allowing your sense of judgment to be controlled by what you feel others think, try it for yourself. There is room for consulting a physician before commencing the blood type diet.

A general test was conducted on 1, 455 adults in the year 2014 to test whether the diet works. It was found type A diet which contains large fruits and veggies showed greater benefits as it affects their health positively.

Supporting the basis for D'Adamo's diet, there are researches that show with evidence that the risk of developing particular diseases differs between different blood types. A study conducted for more than 20 years and published in the year 2012 by the American Heart Association in supporting D' Adamo's postulation stated that blood type O have a low risk of developing heart diseases. That is why D'Adamo is of the view that eating according to your blood type can further your health and result in weight loss. The majority of the people who have tested blood type diet have said that it is beneficial for them.

Furthermore, a study that was published in the year 2007 in lending its support to the diet developed by Naturopath D'Adamo in the Journal of Nutritional and

Environmental Medicine, Dr. Laura Power described the result of her finding that shows allergic reactions to foods on the ground of blood type. The result of her research found that certain responses occur because of blood type, thus justifying D'Adamo's blood type diet. According to the research, those with Rh-negative blood responded most seriously with milk, eggs, cheese, beans, nuts, and gluten.

There are other doctors, such as Doctor Melinda Ratini who have supported D' Adamo's blood type diet. She stated that if you follow this restrictive diet, you will lose weight because you are cutting down on other major food groups.

Even though there are scientific breakthroughs in the blood type diet confirming its efficacy in the medical community, the medical society is still sharply deeply divided. However, you should determine what works for you. Do not base your opinion on what people say. Have you tried it and it failed? It is only your experience with the blood type diet that can give you the confidence to say whether the diet works or not.

This common mistake has been the bane of many dieters.

Mistake # 24: The 100 Metres Dash Race

Clearing your refrigerator, restocking your pantry is a powerful step that people who want to lose weight in the blood type diet have to take. You have done well, and I will say that your efforts are highly commendable. But I am worried about the manner that you go about it. I am worried that your migration is rather too sudden. I am worried about your high speed. I am equally worried about your 100 metres race that you have commenced. I wished you can listen to my advice now and take things slowly. Begin the restocking of your refrigerator, your pantry in a slow manner. There is no need to be hasty. If you race like this when starting the blood type diet, I am afraid that you may soon crash. Give your life and your body the time to adjust gradually. The diet has to be done in a manner that will allow your body the time to adjust. This sounded basic, yet a mistake that can make you stop dieting too early or stop it completely.

Mistake #25: The Journal Accident

I have cautioned about keeping too much eye on the scale, yet you still need to keep a good record of the progress of your weight loss. A blood type diet journal is very consequential. In the blood type diet journal, you will record all the observational changes that you experience in the blood type diet. Record the rate of your weight loss in your journal each time you climb the scale. Note the foods that cause allergy in your body. By keeping account of your weight loss, you are able to better assess your success in the diet. Possessing a blood type diet journal is a valuable record tool for assessing your entire progress in the blood type diet.

THE END

Did you enjoyed this book, I would appreciate if you can take a minute and write a review.

Emily Fan

Other books by the same author

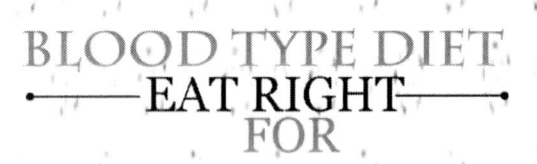

BLOOD TYPE DIET: EAT RIGHT FOR YOUR BLOOD TYPE FOOD AND

SUPPLEMENTS FOR TYPE O - Kindle edition by EMILY FAN.

BLOOD TYPE DIET
EAT RIGHT FOR
YOUR BLOOD TYPE

FOOD AND SUPPLEMENTS FOR TYPE A

A QUICK REFERENCE GUIDE FOR BLOOD TYPE A FOOD AND SUPPLEMENTS

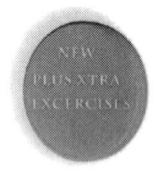

NEW PLUS XTRA EXCERCISES

EMILY FAN

BLOOD TYPE DIET: EAT RIGHT FOR YOUR BLOOD TYPE FOOD AND SUPPLEMENTS FOR TYPE A - Kindle edition by EMILY FAN. Health, Fitness & Dieting Kindle eBooks @ Amazon.com.

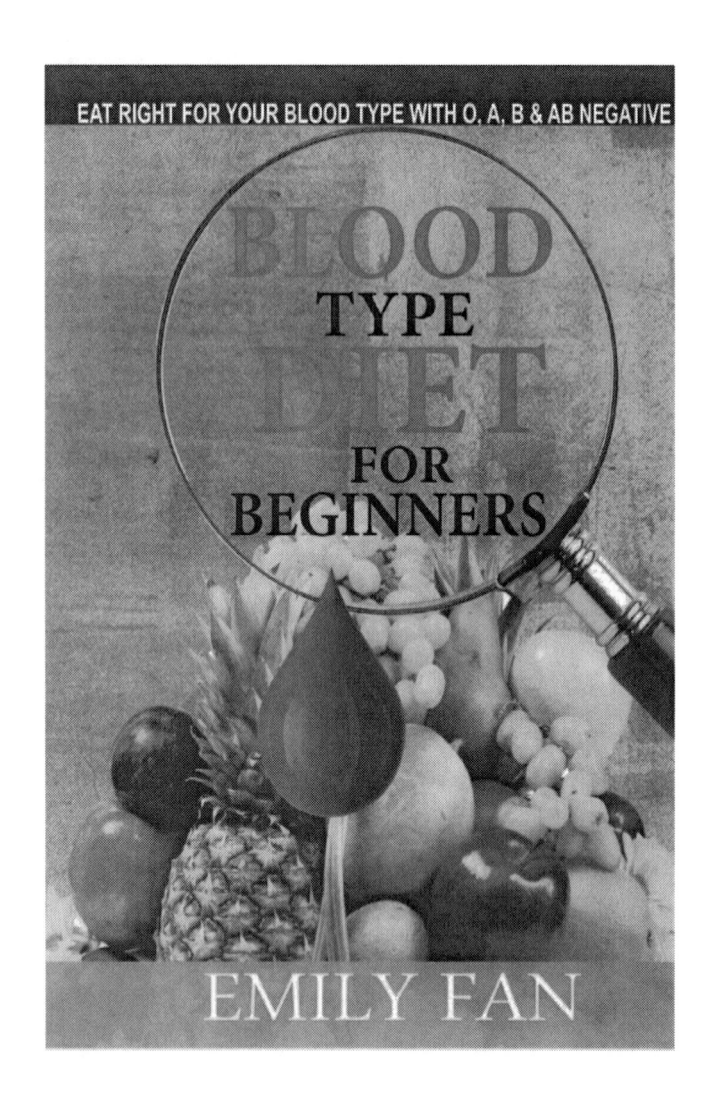

Amazon.com: BLOOD TYPE DIET FOR BEGINNERS: Eat Right For Your Blood

Type With O, A, B And AB Negative eBook:

Emily Fan

BLOOD
TYPE O
Diet

Eating Right For Your Blood Type Recipes that will flavour Your

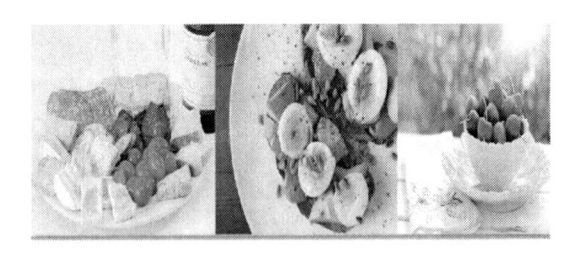

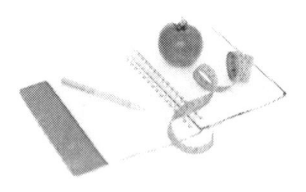

Emily Fan

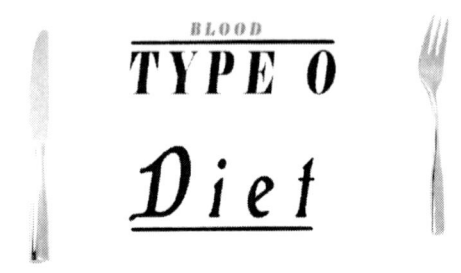

BLOOD TYPE O DIET: EATING RIGHT FOR YOUR BLOOD TYPE RECIPES THAT WILL FLAVOUR YOUR LIFE - Kindle

edition by Emily Fan. Health, Fitness & Dieting Kindle eBooks @ Amazon.com.

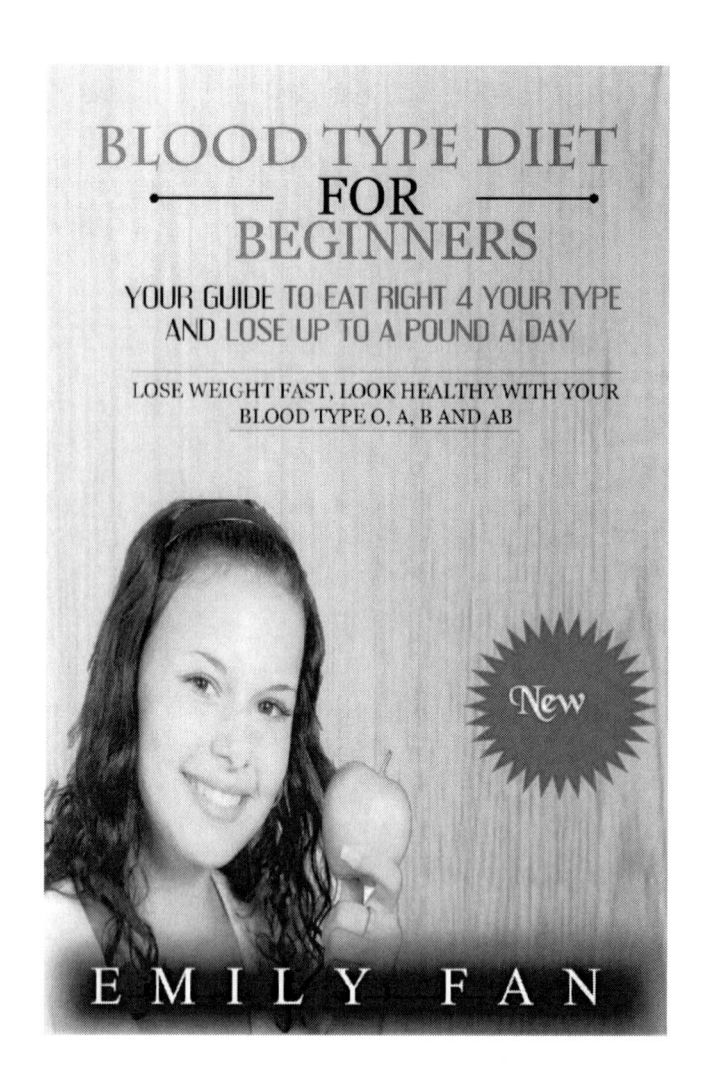

Blood Type Diet Mistakes to Avoid

[Amazon.com: BLOOD TYPE DIET FOR BEGINNERS: Your Guide To Eat Right 4 Your Type And Lose Up To A Pound A Day: Lose Weight Fast, Look Healthy With Your Blood Type O, A, B And AB eBook: EMILY FAN: Kindle Store](#)